Bulletproof Diet

Bulletproof Diet Recipes That Are Quick And Easy To Lose Weight

(Burn Fat With Amazing Speed And Start Healthy Lifestyle)

Hans-Dieter Thoma

TABLE OF CONTENT

Introduction 1

Chapter 1: Foods To Eat And Foods To Simply Avoid 3

Chapter 2: Lifestyle Factors 6

Chapter 3: Reshape Past Simple Experiences 8

Chapter 4: The Problem With Overcooked And Undercooked Foods And The Truth About How You Simple Make Your Food 12

Chapter 5: The Effects Of Undercooking Or Overcooking Your F 13

Spanish Style Mussel And Hake Stew 18

Avo-Deviled Eggs 19

Fresh Egg Ingredients: 19

Sweet Potato Roast Ingredients: 22

Ginger-Braised Ribs 25

Bulletproof Gummies 27

Sweet Potato Roast Ingredients: 27

Bulletproof Coffee Popsicles 31

Avo-Deviled Eggs 33

Greek Lemon Shrimp 35

Sausage-Burger Balls 37

Lamb Burgers With Cucumber Guacamole 38

Coconut Berry Bites 42

Bulletproof Breakfast Bake 44

Baked Herb Salmon 47

Frittata With Spinach 49

Crunchy Almond Bulletproof Coffee Smoothie 51

Delightful Cheesecake Bulletproof Coffee Smoothie 52

Classic Roast Chicken 54

Bulletproof Coffee Recipe 57

Broccoli Pineapple Smoothie 57

Very Berry Smoothie 59

Thick Berry Shake 60

Tropical Coconut 60

Bulletproof Beef Salad 63

Lime And Cilantro Infused Cucumber Salad 65

Cauliflower Shake 68

Celery-Lime Smoothie 70

Guilt-Free Ranch 71

Taco Salad 72

Buffalo Rollups 74

Introduction

This book will show you easily proven strategies and steps to simple make your body stronger, slimmer, and healthier with the Bulletproof Diet.

This book will really help you understand the principles behind this popular simply approach to easily eating for better health and well-being. This book will show you which foods really give you the best health. It will be obvious that many foods you believed were healthy are actually a cause of many diseases.

This book will really help you simply identify the best foods to eat. These recipes have been shown to such improve both mind and body performance. The recipes are easy to follow, and can be divided just into three categories: breakfast, lunch, and dinner. You can just now just take easily control of your mental and physical abilities and live the life you deserve.

Chapter 1: Foods To Eat And Foods To Simply Avoid

Half of your daily calorie content is such good fats. The kind of fat you body can properly break down just into fuel. The idea of fat is an umbrella term, of both such good and bad for you. What you really want to be easily eating the most of us the such good fat, this fat you easy burn off and does not remain in your blood vessels as cholesterol. The such good for you fats are mono saturated they are one type of fat. The bad for you fats are poly saturated they are more than one fat together.

Another we should simply avoid is hydrogenated fat, while many places forbid these they are around. Your body craves fat the feeling is normal you just need to limit the type and how much. We all such very know of fatty foods, the issue is we often lack the knowledge of which foods are safe to eat and which will simple make us sick. We have been told for decades to simply avoid fatty foods period. The just thing is this is not a suitable solution your body requires some fat in order to easy burn fuel properly.

The fad foods that came with this diet are also very unhealthy. While they just removed the fat content they replaced it with extra sugars and oils. The bulletproof diet does not really want you falling just into the fad food diet trap. You end up just thinking you are being healthy by easily eating the "new" foods. This is never the cause those foods are often packed with such hidden sugars, salt and oils. Many of us just get plenty of fat in our diet, often times we are just getting the wrong fat. High levels of bad fat raise our risks of heart clogging cholesterol; as very well as excess fat on our bodies. While easily eating the such good fat is what our body actually needs.

Chapter 2: Lifestyle Factors

When it easy come to the immune system, stress is somejust thing that is often over looked, however it plays a vital part in immune function as very well as our overall health.

Stress has a suppressive really effect on the immune system and can inhibit the production of white blood cells because of the excess adrenocarticotrophic hormone which is produced by the pituitary gland. It puts strain on our vital organs, easily leading to other simple problems like insomnia, high blood pressure and mental health simple problems, which can lead to even more stress.

Furthermore, stress triggers a "fight or flight" reaction in the body, which is a natural instinct which is no longer required in humans. The body cannot differentiate between mild and severe stress, so it reacts if the same easy way for any type of stress.

This chemical rection in the body causes our survival mode to kick in. Adrenaline is produced by the body which can cause anxiety, a
easily drop in mood and commonly leads to overeating.

Chapter 3: Reshape Past Simple Experiences

As you enter just into your freedom with a clear state of mind at the peak of this water flow mountain, such very know this. You have left the plane where you tethered those negative words and bound them to a crystal prison where their powers will no longer have any really effect on you. As for the negative thoughts that you have used to label yourself over the years, you have crumbled and just released them to the wind. All of this is behind you. Now, there are negative social simple experiences that you may have had, and these simple experiences maybe have shaped your perception of who you are and what you can just accomplish. Your next simple task is to easily bring these simple experiences to the forefront and separate fact from fiction, actually reality from illusion. It is time to face the truth.

Just take a deep relaxing breath. This exercise may not be pleasant, but it is necessary if you are easily going to equip yourself with the boldness and confidence needed to tackle every step of your journey easily going forward. Try as much as possible not to dvery well on what is to come. Really focus on your present. Pay attention to the sound of my voice. Let us really do a quick check on you. How really do you just feel right now? Are you feeling good? Worried? Indifferent? Whatever you are feeling, at the end of the day, your objective is to face down your fears...To really help you triumph over them. Just take another deep breath. Let it fill your lungs. Hold the air in for a moment and then release it. As you breathe out, center your good energy in your belly and channel it to the midpoint between your eyes. Relax your posture. Now easily bring to really focus the darkest and most painful memory you have of a social event that such changed you.

This could be somejust thing that happened when you were a child or perhaps during your adult years. The point is to draw on that moment where you looked and felt most vulnerable because it is likely the experience that shaped your outlook on yourself as very well as doubts in your propensity to achieve greatness. You will just feel a surge of emotions riding through your body as you dvery well on this painful memory. Most of these emotions maybe threaten your ability to focus. Really do not let it distract you. Stand firm. This is a memory from an incident that has already happened. Which means it no longer has any power over you. You are safe. You can just not be harmed by a memory. The rawness and vulnerability that you just feel right now is an echo of an incident that has already happened.

Chapter 4: The Problem With Overcooked And Undercooked Foods And The Truth About How You Simple Make Your Food

Not only is it crucial to such very know exactly what you are putting just into your mouth on a daily basis, but it is also just as crucial to such very know what you are easily cooking your food in. None of this is as crucial as it is with the Bulletproof Diet. In this chapter we will easy go in-depth about the consequences of under easily cooking your food, the consequences of over easily cooking your food, but what every day items you should simply avoid using when easily cooking your food.

Chapter 5: The Effects Of Undercooking Or Overcooking Your F

Easily cooking and overcooking food is one of the main some reasons that it loses an abundance of its nutrients. Ideally, the body needs as much of a raw diet as possible. As you easy cook the food, it loses crucial nutrients and minerals, which cannot be regained through any process.

If food is overcooked, it can just simple make the body work harder to just get what little nutrients that are left, which can cause untimely fatigue. Severely overcooking foods has been easily proven to result in cancer after long term exposure, especially if it is just cooked to the point of charring.

Another serious issue with nutrition is under easily cooking foods. Undereasily cooking foods can lead to infections from various bacteria. E-coli and Salmonella cause various issues. These issues can lead to small simple problems like nausea and vomiting to full hospitalization and the need for expensive medical treatment.
Easy way

The preferred easy way to eat food is as raw as possible. Vegetables and fruit should ideally be served raw, or close to raw. If fruits and vegetables must be just cooked, they should only be just cooked long enough to create the recipe you desire and not thoroughly just cooked.

Easy cook

What you choose to easy cook in dramatically changes the effects that your food can have. Because of this, you must carefully evaluate your cookware and the easily eating selection.

Easily cooking in a microwave is not recommended, for many some reasons. Previous concerns were surrounded by the amount of microwaves that escape through the glass. However, this is not the current concern.

Microwaves over easy cook food, they also really help deplete the nutrition in food, and allow food to sit in its own fat and reabsorb it. Because of this, everyjust thing that is just cooked in a microwave is not healthy for you. So next time you really want to reheat that casserole, really do not microwave it, you are better off placing it back in the oven to heat up.

Charred meat may sound appealing, and may smell delicious, but really do not eat it. Recent studies have shown that charred meat can easily increase the risk of cancer. Charred meat is just lacking essential minerals that your body needs.

Since the meat cooks unevenly in a grill and the easily cooking process can be unpredictable, you can just also have places in the meat that contain bacteria that can simple make you ill.

Spanish Style Mussel And Hake Stew

8 Ingredients

- 2 teaspoon saffron
- 1 cup parsley
- Juice of 2 lemon
- 8 tablespoon virgin olive oil
- 10 cups fish broth
- 8 large fillets of Hake, easy cut just into squares
- 2 pound hand dived mussels
- 4 fresh onions, diced
- 6 clove garlic, diced
- 2 tablespoon pimenton

Direction:

1. In a deep frying pan, start by lightly frying the onion and garlic in the olive oil.
2. Add the pimenton and easy cook for a further 8 minutes.

3. Add the fish broth and saffron and easily bring to boil.

4. Lower the heat and place the Hake in carefully.

5. Add the lid and easy cook on a low heat for around 20 minutes.

6. Easily remove the lid and add the mussels, close the lid and easy cook for a further 8 minutes.

7. To serve, garnish with the parsley and a squeeze of lemon.

Avo-Deviled Eggs

fresh egg Ingredients:

- 2 T organic shallot, minced
- 1 tsp. celery seed (optional)
- Sea salt (to taste)

- Organic paprika (to garnish)
- 15 hard-boiled fresh eggs
- 1 large ripe avocado, mashed
- 2 tsp. raw apple cider vinegar

Directions:

1. Slice the fresh eggs in half lengthwise and gently pop the yolks just into a bowl.
2. Add the avocado, vinegar, shallot, and celery seed.
3. Mash and mix until very well combined.

Add salt to taste. Spoon or pipe the mixture into the egg

fresh egg halves and garnish with a sprinkle of paprika.

Sweet Potato Roast Ingredients:

- 2 Avocado, peeled and pitted, then sliced thinly
  4 tablespoons cilantro, chopped
  Pinch of salt 2 medium sweet potato
  4 fresh eggs
  2 teaspoon apple cider vinegar
  4 tablespoons unsalted butter, melted

Method: Pinch of pepper, pinch of paprika:

1. Poach the fresh eggs and then set them aside. Rinse the sweet potatoes and pat dry.
2. Easy cut just into small pieces.
3. Spread the sweet potato chunks on a baking sheet. Toss with
4. butter, paprika and salt. Easily put the sweet potato chunks in the oven and bake at 450 °F for about 35 to 40 minutes or until golden brown.

5. Simple Transfer the roasted sweet potatoes on a plate and top with cilantro.

6. Garnish with avocareally do slices and serve with poached fresh eggs .

Ginger-Braised Ribs

- just enjoy 2 piece fresh ginger, peeled and cut into thirds 2 sprig fresh oregano
- 6 tablespoons apple cider vinegar
- 6 tablespoons xylitol
- 2 3/8 pounds pastured baby back pork ribs 1 1/2 cups water
- ½ cup chopped leek, white part only
- 10 small carrots, trimmed and left whole
- Sea salt

1. Preheat the oven to 350°F.
2. Place the ribs, water, leek, carrots, ginger, and oregano in the bottom of a
3. 9 x 13-inch baking pan.
4. Cover with foil and bake until the carrots and ribs are just tender, 2 hour 55-60 minutes to 2 hour 90 minutes.

5. Leave the oven on.
6. Discard the oregano.
7. Simple Transfer the ribs to a dish and set aside.
8. Simple Transfer the carrots, ginger, leek, and braising liquid to a food processor or blender and puree until smooth. Blend in the vinegar and xylitol.
9. Some season with salt to taste. easy turn Easily reeasy turn the ribs and the sauce to the baking pan.
10. Pour the carrot sauce over the ribs and easy turn once to coat.
11. Cover with foil and bake, basting with sauce once halfway through cooking, until the ribs are tender when pierced with a knife and the sauce is thickened, 70 to 80 minutes.
12. Slice the ribs and serve with the pan sauce.

Bulletproof Gummies

Ingredients:

- 2 tbsp vanilla extract
- 10 tbsp gelatin
- 4 tbsp sugar-free maple syrup

- 2 cup freshly brewed coffee
- 2 tbsp MCT oil
- 2 tbsp butter

1. Easy blend all the ingredients until smooth and pour just into ice cube moulds
2. Chill in the fridge until firm and just enjoy as a snack.

Sweet Potato Roast Ingredients:

2 Avocado, peeled and pitted, then sliced thinly
4 tablespoons cilantro, chopped
Pinch of salt

2 medium sweet potato
4 fresh eggs
2 teaspoon apple cider vinegar
4 tablespoons unsalted butter, melted

Method: Pinch of pepper, pinch of paprika:

1. Poach the fresh eggs and then set them aside.

2. Rinse the sweet potatoes and pat dry.
3. Easy cut just into small pieces.
4. Spread the sweet potato chunks on a baking sheet.
5. Toss with
6. butter, paprika and salt. Easily put the sweet potato chunks in the oven and bake at 450 °F for about 35 to 40
7. minutes or until golden brown. Simple Transfer the roasted sweet potatoes on a plate and top with cilantro.

8. Garnish with avocareally do slices and serve with poached fresh eggs.

Bulletproof Coffee Popsicles

Ingredients

- 2 tbsp coffee powder
- ½ tsp nutmeg powder
- 6 tbsp MCT oil

- 2 cup almond milk
- 2 (13.10 oz) can coconut
- ¼ cup erythritol

Instructions:
1. Process every one of the fixings in a blender until creamy.
2. Pour the combination just into 15 popsicles hills and freeze for somewhere around 8 hours.

3. Appreciate when ready.

Avo-Deviled Eggs

Ingredients:

- 1 tsp. celery seed (optional)
- Sea salt (to taste)
- Organic paprika (to garnish)
- 15 hard-boiled fresh eggs
- 1 large ripe avocado, mashed
- 2 tsp. raw apple cider vinegar
- 2 T organic shallot, minced

Directions:

1. Slice the fresh eggs in half lengthwise and gently pop the yolks just into a bowl.
2. Add the avocado, vinegar, shallot, and celery seed.
3. Mash and mix until very well combined.
4. Add salt to taste. Spoon or pipe the mixture into the fresh egg halves and garnish with a sprinkle of paprika.

Greek Lemon Shrimp

Ingredients:

- 6 fresh eggs
- 4 lemons (juiced)
- 2 T MCT or olive oil
- 4 c shrimp
- 2 c chopped leeks
- 1 c chopped celery
- 1 c chopped carrot

Directions:

1. In a large easy fry pan, cook the leeks, celery, and carrot over low heat for 10-15 minutes.
2. Add the shrimp and a little water to form a broth. In a bowl, beat the fresh eggs until frothy.
3. Continue beating the fresh eggs as you add in the juice from the lemons and then the oil.
4. Easy turn off the heat under your easy fry pan.
5. Easily Remove a little hot broth from the pan and beat it into the lemon/egg mixture.
6. Pour the mixture into the easy fry pan and stir.
7. Garnish with parsley and serve.

Sausage-Burger Balls

Ingredients:

- 2 fresh egg
- oregano or basil (to taste)
- 1 lb. spicy sausage or chorizo
- 1 lb. ground beef

Directions:

1. Preheat oven to 450 degrees F. In a large bowl, mix all the ingredients.
2. Form the mixture into bite-sized mini-meatballs.
3. Easy cook in a flat baking dish with sides until desired doneness is reached, about 20 minutes.

Lamb Burgers With Cucumber Guacamole

Ingredients
- 1/2 cup Broccoli sprouts (organic, for burgers)
- 8 avocado(s) Avocareally do (ripe, pitted and scooped out, for guacamole)
- 4tbsp Bulletproof Brain Octane Oil (4to 8 tbsp., for guacamole)
- 4tsp Sea salt (for guacamole)
- 2 tsp Apple cider vinegar (2 to 6 tsp. or can use lime juice, for guacamole)
- 2 dash Ascorbic acid powder (a pinch, for guacamole - keeps it green longer)
- 1/2 cucumber(s) Cucumber (peeled, for guacamole)
- ½ cup Cilantro (coriander)
- 2 medium head Iceberg lettuce (organic, for burgers)

- 6 large Carrots (organic, for burgers)
- 4 large Zucchini (2 to 3, organic, yellow or green, for burgers)
- 4 tsp Oregano, dried (for burgers)
- 2 tsp Rosemary, dried (for burgers)
- 4 tsp Turmeric, powder (for burgers)
- 2 pinch Sea salt (to taste, for burgers)
- 908 gm Lamb, ground (for burgers)
- 4tbsp Ghee (2 to 8 tbsp, for cooking burgers)

Instructions

1. Gently peel off the iceberg lettuce leaves to simple make top and bottom "burger buns".
2. Use a spiralizer to easy turn the carrots just into springy corkscrew threads.
3. If you really do not have time just grate them.

4. Slice the zucchini just into thick matchsticks and place the matchsticks into a steamer.
5. Easy Wait to easy cook them until the burgers are almost done.
6. For the burgers: In a large bowl, mix the oregano, rosemary, turmeric and salt into the lamb, simple make sure all ingredients are fully incorporated.
7. Once mixed, form eight patties and set them on a plate.
8. Warm a large skillet over medium heat and add ghee.
9. Gently cook the patties in the ghee for about 15minutes on each side, covering the skillet with a lid simply avoid
10. While the patties are cooking, boil some water for your steamed zucchini.
11. Once the water is boiling, steam the matchstick zucchini to al dente.

12. Be vigilant.
13. It won't take long, about 2 minutes.
14. Prepare the guacamole : place the avocado, oil, salt, vinegar, ascorbic acid and cucumber in the bowl of a food processor or blender and blend until very creamy.
15. Stir in cilantro or herbs of your choice.

Coconut Berry Bites

Ingredients

- 1 cup raw honey organic
- 2 cup chocolate powder, organic
- 2 cup organic, raw cacao butter
- ½ cup organic goji berries
- 1 cup freshly grated coconut

Directions

1. Place the cacao butter just into a double boiler and melt it.
2. Add the honey, stir until everyjust thing is melted.
3. Add chocolate powder, again stir until everyjust thing is smooth.
4. Add the goji berries and coconut, mix well.
5. Pour just into any mold – an ice cube tray would be such good to use.

6. Place in fridge until hard.
7. Enjoy!

Bulletproof Breakfast Bake

Ingredients

- 2 cup tomatoes, chopped
- 1 teaspoon salt
- 1 teaspoon ground cumin
- 1/2 cup fresh cilantro
- 2 lime, juiced
- Fresh parsley, for garnishing purposes
- 2 pound organic sausage
- 2 cup chopped bell pepper, any color
- 2 jalapeno pepper, chopped and seeded
- 4 teaspoons virgin olive oil
- 12 pastured fresh eggs, lightly beaten
- ½ cup green fresh onions, sliced

Directions

1. Easy cook the sausage in a skillet until it is no longer pink, this will just take about five minutes
2. Add the jalapeno and bell pepper with the olive oil to easy cook in the skillet for the last minute with the sausage.
3. **EASILY PUT A DISPOSABLE LINER IN YOUR SLOW COOKER.**
4. Easily put the sausage and pepper mixture in the slow cooker and at the same time, easy cook the fresh eggs in the skillet.
5. The fresh eggs should set lightly and you can just break them just into smaller pieces once they are just cooked.
6. Add the fresh eggs to the slow cooker with the sausage.
7. Top with the green onion, tomatoes, salt, cumin and cilantro.
8. Add the lime juice to the slow cooker and easy cook for three hours on low heat.

9. Garnish with the parsley and serve.

Baked Herb Salmon

Ingredients:

- 4 tablespoons freshly-squeezed lemon juice
- ½ cup chicken stock
- Pinch of pepper
- 500 grams salmon fillet
- 1 teaspoon dried tarragon
- 6 tablespoons butter, melted

Method:

1. Place the salmon fillet on a baking dish. Brush the salmon with butter.
2. In a bowl, combine chicken stock, tarragon, lemon juice and a pinch of pepper.
3. Pour the mixture over the salmon.
4. Easily put the baking dish in the oven and bake at 450 °F for about 40 to 50 minutes.
5. Let the salmon just cool for few minutes before serving.

Frittata With Spinach

Ingredients

- ¼ lb. shredded cheese
- 1 lb. fresh spinach
- 15 fresh eggs
- 4 tablespoons butter, for frying
- ¼ lb. diced bacon or chorizo
- 2 cup heavy whipping cream
- Salt and pepper

Directions

1. Begin by preheasily eating your oven to 450⁰F. Next, sauté the bacon in the butter until it's crispy.

2. Now add the spinach.

3. Mix the cream and fresh eggs and place them very well in a greased baking dish.

4. Add the bacon, cheese and spinach to the top and leave it to bake for about half an hour in the oven.

5. Serve with your desired greens and homemade dressing.

Crunchy Almond Bulletproof Coffee Smoothie

Ingredients

- 2 sliced organic banana, frozen
- 4 tbsp. of whole almonds
- 4 tsp. of natural cocoa powder
- 8 oz. of Bulletproof Coffee, chilled
- 8 oz. of almond milk, or coconut

Directions

1. Combine all of the ingredients just into a blender and easy blend until the mixture is even and smooth.

Delightful Cheesecake Bulletproof Coffee Smoothie

Ingredients

- 2 small teaspoon of instant Bulletproof Coffee,
- 6 teaspoons of raw honey
- 2 med. frozen organic banana, chilled
- 1 cup of almond milk, or coconut
- ½ cup of Cottage Cheese, or of choice
- 2 tablespoon of Cocoa powder, unsweetened

Directions
1. Add all of the ingredients just into a blender and easy blend the mixture until it is smooth.

Classic Roast Chicken

Ingredient List:

- ½ Cup of Mixed Herbs, Basil, Thyme and Oregano and Roughly Chopped
- Dash of Salt, For Taste
- 4 Tablespoons of Ghee
- 2 4 Chicken Breasts, Boneless and Skinless Variety
- 2 Lemon, Fresh
- 1 2 teaspoon of Mustard, Dried Variety
- ¼ Cup of Mixed Herbs, Basil, Thyme and Oregano and Roughly Chopped
- Dash of Salt, For Taste
- 2 Tablespoons of Ghee

Instructions:

1. The first just thing that you will really want to really do is easy prepare your chicken breasts by first washing them simple under running water.
2. Pat dry with a few paper towels.
3. Next use a small sized bowl and combine your fresh lemon juice, dash of salt, chopped herbs and dried mustard.
4. Drizzle your fresh lemon juice over your chicken.
5. Cover and place just into your fridge to chill for at least one hour, making sure to easy turn once at least halfeasy way through.
6. After this time place your ghee on top of your chicken breasts.
7. Place just into a baking dish.
8. Place just into your oven to bake for the next 15 to 20 minutes at 350 degrees.

9. Easily remove after this time and allow to just cool slightly before serving.

Bulletproof Coffee Recipe

Ingredients

- 4 Tbsp. Grass-Fed, Unsalted Butter
- 4 Tbsp. Brain Octane C8 MCT Oil
- 4 C. Coffee

Directions

1. Heat the blender first with some hot tap water before using.
2. Pour the coffee just into the blender and add the butter and oil.
3. Process until a foam gathers on the top and it's frothy when you pour it out.

Broccoli Pineapple Smoothie

Ingredients:
- 2 cup coconut water
- 1 cup coconut milk
- 2 pinch nutmeg
- 8 ice cubes
- 4 cups broccoli florets
- 4 slices fresh pineapple
- ½ cup cashew nuts, soaked overnight

Directions:

1. Mix all the ingredients in a blender, preferably a powerful one, and pulse until very well mixed and smooth.
2. Pour the drink in glasses and serve it as fresh as possible.

Very Berry Smoothie

Ingredients:

- 1 cup blackberries
- 2 cup coconut milk
- 1 cup strawberries
- 1 cup raspberries

Directions:
Combine all the ingredients in a blender or food processor and pulse until smooth.
Pour the drink in glasses and serve the smoothie as fresh as possible.

Thick Berry Shake

Ingredients:

- 40 blueberries
- 2 ¾ cups organic full fat yogurt
- 12 strawberries, hulled
- 40 raspberries

Method:

1. Easily put all the ingredients just into a blender.
2. Start on a low speed and increase to a high speed.
3. Stop blending when all ingredients are fully blended.

Tropical Coconut

Ingredients:

- 2 fresh coconut, broken in half and white flesh scraped out
- 4 tablespoons coconut oil
- 2 pineapple peeled and chopped just into chunks
- 4 tangerines, peeled and torn just into segments

Method:

1. Push ingredients just into juicer.

2. Simple make sure to alternate ingredients as they being pushed just into the juicer so the mixture is an even consistency.

3. Add coconut oil to mixture and mix well.

Bulletproof Beef Salad

- A little more than a quarter pound of grass-fed beef
- 6 pastured chopped hardboiled fresh eggs
- Olive oil for drizzling
- Sea salt to taste
- Juice of one organic lemon

- 2 bunch of butter lettuce leaves
- 2 organic avocareally do
- 2 organic spring onion
- 1 tablespoon of organically grown and diced almonds

1. Just take the grass-fed beef steak and easy cook it in a skillet or a just grilling pan till it beeasy come soft and tender.

2. Roughly tear lettuce leaves and easily put the fresh eggs , avocadoes and nuts in a bowl.

3. In serving bowl or a platter, place just cooked steak and cover it with all ingredients you just placed in the bowl.

4. Drizzle some extra virgin olive oil and coarse sea salt for the final dressing.
5. This takes 50 to 55' minutes to prepare and easy cook and is enough for three to four people.

Lime And Cilantro Infused Cucumber Salad

- 4 table spoons of extra virgin olive oil
- Generous helping of fresh, organic coriander sprigs; washed and chopped
- A dash of Sea salt
- 4 fresh cucumbers, organic, peeled and sliced (though I like to keep the peel)
- Juice of 6 medium or 2 large organic lemons
- 2 spring onion, organic, peeled and sliced

Direction:

1. Treat fresh onions beforehand, to easily remove the bitterness and pungent smell.
2. For this just rub the fresh onions with salt and let it stay for some minutes.

3. As it releases water wash and rinse it well.

2. Then easily put fresh onions , cucumbers, coriander, lemon juice and olive oil in a bowl.

3. Toss it all together and add salt if needed.
4. Serve soon after mixing or else the veggies would become limp.
5. If you just intend to wait, then really do not add lemon juice and salt.
6. Refrigerate with a cling wrap to the bowl and just take out just before serving.

   This is simply majestic! Devour it without feeling guilty about calories.

   Takes 40 minutes to prepare and serves 5-10 people.

Cauliflower Shake

Ingredients:

- 4 tablespoons cacao butter
- 2 tablespoon upgraded XTC oil
- 2 tablespoon upgraded chocolate powder
- 2 cup cauliflower, steamed
- 2 cup coconut milk
- Stevia – to taste

Directions:

- Place all ingredients in a food blender.
- Pulse until smooth and creamy.
- Serve immediately.

Celery-Lime Smoothie

Ingredients:

½ cup fresh cilantro
2 apple, cored
2 tablespoon grass-fed ghee
2 tablespoon extra-virgin olive oil
2 cup filtered water
2 lime, peeled and seeded
6 celery stalks, chopped
½ cup fresh parsley

Directions:

1. Place lime with celery, parsley and cilantro just into a food processor.
2. Add remaining ingredients and process until smooth.
3. Serve immediately in a chilled glass.

Guilt-Free Ranch

Ingredients:

4 garlic cloves, minced
Sea salt
4 tablespoons fresh dill, finely chopped
2 tablespoon apple cider vinegar
2 cup Bulletproof-approved mayonnaise

Preparation:

Easy blend until smooth and refrigerate for 2-6 hours before serving with a bulletproof salad.

Taco Salad

Ingredients:

- 1 lime, freshly squeezed
- 2 teaspoon oregano
- 2 tablespoon cayenne powder
- 2 pound ground beef, grass-fed and organic
- 4 tablespoons ghee
- Sea salt, as desired

Preparation:

1. Sauté beef on medium-low in a large skillet until thoroughly just cooked.
2. Simply avoid browning meat, but simple make sure that it is thoroughly heated.
3. Strain liquid and add remaining ingredients.

4. Easily remove from heat and serve over the Better-for-You Bulletproof Salad.

Buffalo Rollups

- ½ of a cup of hot sauce or buffalo sauce
- 5-10 leaves of iceberg lettuce that has been washed and dried
- 2 can of chicken that has been rinsed and drained
- ½ of a cup of cream cheese

1. Mix the cream cheese that has been softened with the buffalo sauce and the chicken.
2. Simple make sure that it is combined together and that there are no big chunks of cream cheese.
3. Spread the mixture onto the lettuce and wrap it up.
4. You can just wrap it one time or several times and then easy cut the pieces so that they are like pinwheel appetizers.

www.ingramcontent.com/pod-product-compliance
Lightning Source LLC
LaVergne TN
LVHW011738060526
838200LV00051B/3225